GLUTEN-FREE COOKBOOK FOR SENIORS

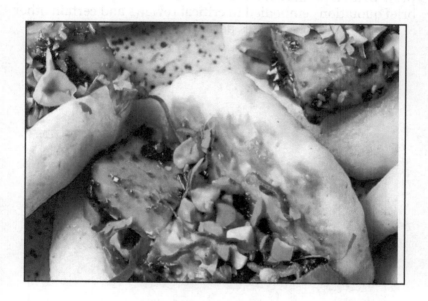

The Complete and Easy Guide to Gluten-free Recipes and Meal Plan For the Elderly

MALONEY DEAN

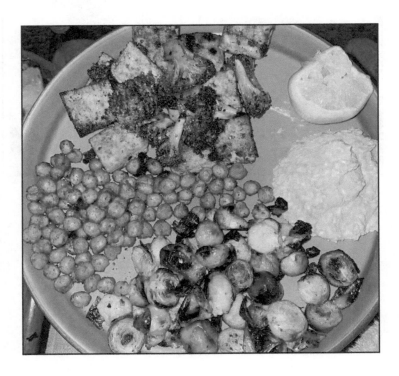

TABLE OF CONTENTS

INTRODUCTION

You are what you eat!!!

This powerful quote became real in the life of a 65-year-old retiree from San Jose, California. This is the tale of a man who, in spite of everything, changed his life by adhering to the straightforward but important gluten-free eating guidelines.

His story not only demonstrates the healing power of food, but it also serves as motivation for senior citizens who want to live longer, healthier lives.

In his mid-60s, John, a retired surveyor, has been battling with high blood pressure, type 2 diabetes, and was at the verge of obesity. His vitality was at an all-time low, and happiness appeared to be a thing of the past.

It was in this depressing and frustrating period that John learned about the idea of a plant-based, gluten-free diet.

As he embarked on this new dietary journey, John noticed a dramatic but steady change. His energy levels and general well-being significantly improved within weeks of switching to a gluten-free diet.

His blood sugar levels returned to normal, and he became less and less dependent on medication. The diet, which was centered on whole, unprocessed foods, opened his eyes to a hitherto undiscovered world of tastes and nutrients.

More than just a list of gluten-free recipes, the foods in this cookbook are a reflection of John's quest for better health. Seniors have been the primary focus of each recipe's creation, with an emphasis on flavor, ease of preparation, and nutritional content.

These meals are intended to keep elders feeling their best all the time, as well as to minimize stress, maintain a healthy stomach, and regulate the immune system.

Those who are experiencing the symptoms of diabetes and High Blood Pressure will find John's story extremely helpful. The meals are carefully balanced to help control blood sugar levels and lower the risk of complications from diabetes.

This is a lifestyle shift, not simply a diet, that enables seniors to take charge of their health and fully enjoy their golden years.

GLUTEN-FREE DIET RECIPES

EXCITING BREAKFAST RECIPES

1. Almond Flour Pancakes

Prep Time: 10 mins
Cook Time: 15 mins
Servings: 4

Ingredients:
1 cup almond flour
2 eggs
1/2 cup almond milk
1 tsp baking powder
2 tbsp honey
1 tsp vanilla extract
Pinch of salt
Coconut oil for cooking

Directions:

Combine almond flour, baking powder, and salt in a bowl.

In another dish, whisk together eggs, almond milk, honey, and vanilla.

Mix the components (Both the dry and wet ingredients).

In a frying pan over medium heat, preheat the coconut oil.

Pour mixture into pancake molds, cook until bubbles appear, and then turn.

Warm up and serve.

Nutritional fact (per serving):

215 calories

50 milligrams of sodium

Potassium: 135 mg

8g of protein

120 milligrams of phosphorus

2. Chia Seed Pudding

Prep Time: 5 mins (plus overnight soaking)

Cook Time: 0 mins

Servings: 2

Ingredients:

1/4 cup chia seeds

1 cup unsweetened almond milk

1 tbsp maple syrup

1/2 tsp vanilla extract

Fresh berries for topping

Directions:

In a bowl, mix together chia seeds, almond milk, vanilla, and maple syrup.

Give it a good stir, then chill for the night.

Top with fresh berries and serve.

Nutritional facts (per serving):

180 calories

30 milligrams of sodium

200 milligrams of potassium

5g of protein

3. Gluten-Free Oatmeal

Prep Time: 5 mins

Cook Time: 10 mins

Servings: 2

Ingredients:

1 cup gluten-free rolled oats

2 cups water or almond milk

Pinch of salt

1 tablespoon honey or maple syrup

1/2 teaspoon cinnamon

Fresh fruit and nuts for topping

Directions:

In a saucepan, mix oats, water (or almond milk), and a small teaspoon of salt.

After bringing to a boil, lower the heat, and simmer for ten minutes while stirring now and then.

Add cinnamon and honey (or maple syrup) and stir.

Top with nuts and fresh fruit.

Nutritional Facts (per serving):

150 calories

20 milligrams of sodium

105 milligrams of potassium

4g of protein

120 milligrams of phosphorus

4. Avocado Toast on Gluten-Free Bread

Prep Time: 5 mins

Cook Time: 5 mins

Servings: 2

Ingredients:

2 slices of gluten-free bread

1 ripe avocado

Lemon juice

Salt and pepper to taste

Red pepper flakes (optional)

Directions:

Toast slices of gluten-free bread until desired crispness is achieved.

Add salt, pepper, and lemon juice to mashed avocado.

Drizzle the avocado mixture over the toast.

If desired, top with red pepper flakes.

Nutritional facts (per serving):

250 calories

200 milligrams of sodium

500 milligrams of potassium

4g of protein

60 milligrams of phosphorus

5. Berry Yogurt Smoothie

Prep Time: 5 mins

Cook Time: 0 mins

Servings: 2

Ingredients:

1 cup mixed berries (fresh or frozen)

1 cup Greek yogurt (gluten-free)

1/2 cup almond milk

1 tbsp honey

Directions:

In a blender, combine berries, yogurt, almond milk, and honey.

Blend till smooth.

Serve right away.

Nutritional Facts (per serving):

145 calories

45 milligrams of sodium

180 milligrams of potassium

8g of protein

100 milligrams of phosphorus

6. Gluten-Free Breakfast Burrito

Prep Time: 15 mins

Cook Time: 10 mins

Servings: 2

Ingredients:

2 gluten-free tortillas

4 eggs

1/2 cup diced bell peppers

1/4 cup shredded cheese (optional)

Salt and pepper to taste

Salsa for serving

Directions:

Add bell peppers, salt, and pepper to scrambled eggs.

As directed on the package, warm the tortillas.

Spoon scrambled eggs into tortillas and sprinkle cheese on top.

Form into burritos and present alongside salsa.

Nutritional Facts (per serving):

320 calories

400 mg of sodium

Potassium: 220 mg

16g of protein

180 milligrams of phosphorus

7. Gluten-Free Veggie Omelette

Prep Time: 10 mins

Cook Time: 10 mins

Servings: 2

Ingredients:

4 eggs

1/4 cup diced tomatoes

1/4 cup chopped spinach

1/4 cup diced mushrooms

1/4 cup shredded cheese (optional)

Salt and pepper to taste

1 tablespoon of olive oil

Directions:

Whisk eggs in a dish. Add pepper and salt for seasoning.

Olive oil is heated in a skillet. Sauté the mushrooms, spinach, and tomatoes.

Spread eggs over vegetables, allow to set, then fold in half and top with cheese.

Serve after the cheese has melted.

Nutritional Facts (per serving):

220 calories

310 mg of sodium

300 milligrams of potassium

14g of protein

200 milligrams of phosphorus

8. Banana Almond Muffins (Gluten-Free)

Prep Time: 15 mins

Cook Time: 20 mins

Servings: 6 muffins

Ingredients:

1 cup almond flour

2 ripe bananas, mashed

1/4 cup maple syrup

2 eggs

1 tsp baking powder

1/2 tsp vanilla extract

Pinch of salt

Directions:

Set the oven temperature to 175°C/350°F. Use paper liners to line a muffin tray.

In a bowl, stir together almond flour, baking powder, and salt.

Beat the eggs, vanilla, maple syrup, and mashed bananas together in a separate bowl.

Mix the components (dry and wet). Transfer to muffin tins.

Remove the toothpick after 20 minutes of baking.

Nutritional Facts (per Serving):

180 calories

80 mg of sodium

150 milligrams of potassium

5g of protein

100 milligrams of phosphorus

9. Quinoa Breakfast Bowl

Prep Time: 5 mins

Cook Time: 20 mins

Servings: 2

Ingredients:

1/2 cup quinoa

1 cup water

1/4 cup almond milk

1 tbsp honey

Fresh fruit for topping

A sprinkle of cinnamon

Directions:

Wash the quinoa in cool water.

Add the quinoa and water to a saucepan. After bringing to a boil, simmer for 15 minutes.

Add honey and almond milk and stir. Simmer for an additional five minutes.

Garnish with a dash of cinnamon and some fresh fruit.

Nutritional Facts (per serving):

210 calories

30 milligrams of sodium

Potassium: 220 mg

6g of protein

170 mg of phosphorus

10. Sweet Potato and Kale Hash

Prep Time: 10 mins

Cook Time: 15 mins

Servings: 2

Ingredients:

1 large sweet potato, diced

1 cup chopped kale

1/2 onion, diced

2 cloves garlic, minced

2 tbsp olive oil

Salt and pepper to taste

1/4 tsp paprika

Directions:

Olive oil is heated in a skillet. Add the onion and sweet potato, and simmer until softened.

Add the paprika, garlic, greens, salt, and pepper. Sauté the kale until it wilts.

Warm up the food.

Nutritional Facts (per serving):

200 calories

70 mg of sodium

400 milligrams of potassium

3g of protein

90 milligrams of phosphorus

TANTALIZING LUNCH RECIPES

11. *Quinoa Vegetable Salad*

Prep Time: 15 minutes

Cooking Time: 20 minutes

Servings: 4

Ingredients:

1 cup quinoa

2 cups water

1 bell pepper, diced

1 cucumber, diced

1/4 cup red onion, finely chopped

1/4 cup olive oil

2 tablespoons lemon juice

Salt and pepper to taste

DIRECTIONS:

Run cold water over the quinoa. Bring the water and quinoa to a boil in a saucepan. For fifteen minutes, simmer, covered, and reduce heat. Give it time to cool.

Combine the chilled quinoa, bell pepper, cucumber, and red onion in a big bowl.

Mix the olive oil, lemon juice, salt, and pepper in a small bowl. Drizzle the salad with the dressing and mix well.

Nutritional Facts:

220 calories

Ten milligrams of sodium

320 milligrams of potassium

Six grams of protein

150 milligrams of phosphorus

12. *Broccoli and Cheese Baked Potato*

Prep Time: 10 minutes

Cooking Time: 1 hour

Servings: 2

Ingredients:

2 large baking potatoes

1 cup broccoli florets

1/2 cup shredded cheddar cheese

1 tablespoon butter

Salt and pepper to taste

Directions:

Oven temperature should be set to 400°F (200°C).

Use a fork to pierce the potatoes, then bake for one hour, or until soft.

To make broccoli florets tender, steam them.

Make a cut on the upper part of every potato.

Using a fork, fluff the insides and stir in the butter, salt, and pepper.

Top with steamed broccoli and in addition to shredded cheese.

Nutritional facts:

300 calories

200 milligrams of sodium

900 milligrams of potassium

12 g of protein

180 milligrams of phosphorus

13. *Avocado with Chicken Wrap*

Prep Time: 20 minutes

Ten minutes for cooking

4 servings

Ingredients:

Two cups of cooked, shredded chicken

Mash two ripe avocados.

half a cup of Greek yogurt

Four tortillas without gluten

One cup of shredded lettuce

To taste, add salt and pepper.

Directions:

Combine Greek yogurt, mashed avocado, and shredded chicken in a bowl. Add pepper and salt for seasoning.

After arranging the tortillas, divide the chicken mixture among them equally.

After adding the shredded lettuce, roll the tortillas.

Nutritional Facts:

350 calories

300 mg of sodium

500 milligrams of potassium

25 g of protein

250 milligrams of phosphorus

14. Tomato-Basil Soup

Prep Time: 10 Minutes

30 minutes for cooking

servings: 4

Ingredients:

Each can is 14.5 oz. chopped tomatoes

One sliced onion

Two minced garlic cloves

Two cups of broth made of vegetables

1/4 cup finely chopped fresh basil

One-fourth cup of heavy cream

Two teaspoon olive oil

To taste, add salt and pepper.

Direction:

Warm up the olive oil in a big pot over medium heat. Add the onion and garlic and cook until tender.

Add the veggie broth and tomatoes. Bring to a boil, then simmer for 20 minutes on low heat.

Add heavy cream and basil. Puree the soup with an immersion blender until it's smooth.

Add pepper and salt for seasoning.

Nutritional facts:

150 calories

410 milligrams of sodium

450 milligrams of potassium

3 g of protein

70 milligrams of phosphorus

15. Spinach and Feta Stuffed Chicken

Prep Time: 15 minutes

25 minutes for cooking

4 servings

Ingredients:

Four skinless and boneless chicken breasts

One cup of chopped spinach and half a cup of crumbled feta cheese

One minced garlic clove and two tablespoons of olive oil

To taste, add salt and pepper.

Directions:

Set the oven to 375°F, or 190°C.

In each chicken breast, make a pocket. Pack with garlic, feta cheese, and spinach.

Use salt and pepper to season the chicken. Heat the olive oil in a skillet over medium heat and brown the chicken on both sides.

After placing in the oven, roast the chicken for 20 minutes or until it is thoroughly done.

Nutritional Facts:

280 calories

400 mg of sodium

500 milligrams of potassium

38 g of protein

300 mg of phosphorus

16. *Grilled Vegetable Platter*

Prep Time: 15 minutes

20 minutes for cooking

servings: 4

Ingredients

One sliced zucchini

One yellow squash, sliced One red bell pepper, sliced

One sliced eggplant

One-fourth cup olive oil

Half a teaspoon balsamic vinegar

To taste, add salt and pepper.

Directions:

Grill at a medium-high temperature.

Combine the vegetables, balsamic vinegar, olive oil, salt, and pepper in a big bowl.

To make veggies soft and slightly browned, grill them for ten minutes, flipping them over one or twice.

Nutritional Facts:

120 calories

30 milligrams of sodium

450 milligrams of potassium

3 g of protein

50 milligrams of phosphorus

17. *Mango and Shrimp Salad*

Prep Time: 20 minutes

Five minutes for cooking

Servings: 4

Ingredients

One pound of peeled and deveined shrimp and one chopped ripe mango

one chopped avocado

1/4 cup of coarsely chopped red onion

1/4 cup finely chopped cilantro

Juice of 1 Lime

Two tsp olive oil

To taste, add salt and pepper.

Directions:

Heat the olive oil in a pan over medium heat. Add the shrimp and simmer for about 5 minutes, or until pink. Allow to cool.

The cooled shrimp, mango, avocado, red onion, and cilantro should all be combined in a big bowl.

After adding a squeeze of lime juice, season with salt and pepper.

Gently toss.

Nutritional Facts:

250 calories

180 milligrams of sodium

400 milligrams of potassium

20 g of protein

220 milligrams of phosphorus

18. *Turkey and Cranberry Salad*

Prep Time: 15 minutes

Cooking Time: 0 minutes

Servings: 4

Ingredients:

2 cups cooked turkey, chopped

1/2 cup dried cranberries

1/2 cup celery, chopped

1/4 cup mayonnaise

1/4 cup Greek yogurt

Salt and pepper to taste

Directions:

Combine turkey, cranberries, and celery in a large bowl.

Mix the Greek yogurt and mayonnaise in a small bowl.

Coat by tossing with the turkey mixture after adding.

Add pepper and salt for seasoning.

Nutritional Facts:

230 calories

190 mg of sodium

300 milligrams of potassium

25 g of protein

200 milligrams of phosphorus

19. Quinoa and Black Bean Salad

Prep Time: 15 minutes

20 minutes for cooking

Servings: 4

Ingredients:

One cup of quinoa

two cups of water

One can of washed and drained black beans

One diced red bell pepper and one-fourth cup of fresh cilantro

Two tsp olive oil

Juice of 1 Lime

To taste, add salt and pepper.

Directions:

Wash the quinoa in cool water. Heat the water in a pot until it boils. For fifteen minutes, cook the quinoa, cover, and lower the heat.

Once the quinoa is fluffy, let it to cool.

Quinoa, black beans, bell pepper, and cilantro should all be combined in a big bowl.

Mix the olive oil, lime juice, salt, and pepper in a small bowl. Add dressing to salad and stir.

Nutritional Facts:

220 calories

15 milligrams of sodium

400 milligrams of potassium

8g of protein

150 milligrams of phosphorus

20. Quinoa Stuffed Peppers with Vegetables

Prep Time: 20 Minutes

40 minutes for cooking

Servings: 4

Ingredients

Four bell peppers, seeded and cut in half

One cup of rinsed quinoa and two cups of veggie broth

One zucchini, one chopped carrot, one chopped onion, two minced garlic cloves, and one tsp olive oil

To taste, add salt and pepper.

Directions:

Set the oven to 375°F, or 190°C.

Bring the vegetable broth and quinoa to a boil in a saucepan. For fifteen minutes, simmer, covered, and reduce heat.

In olive oil, sauté the zucchini, carrot, onion, and garlic until they become soft.

Combine the vegetables and cooked quinoa. Add pepper and salt for seasoning.

Place the quinoa mixture inside the pepper halves.

Bake peppers for 25 minutes, or until soft.

Nutritional Facts:

Sodium: 150 mg

Potassium: 450 mg

Protein: 6 g

Phosphorus: 120 mg

21. *Baked Salmon with Herb Crust*

Prep Time: 10 minutes

Cooking Time: 20 minutes

Servings: 4

Ingredients:
4 salmon fillets

1 tablespoons of olive oil

1/2 cup gluten-free breadcrumbs

2 tablespoons of chopped fresh parsley

1 tablespoon of chopped fresh dill

1 lemon, zest only

Salt and pepper to taste

Directions:
Turn the oven on to 400°F, or 200°C.

Salmon fillets should be put on a baking pan.

Apply a thin layer of olive oil.

Mix the breadcrumbs, dill, parsley, and lemon zest in a bowl.

Add pepper and salt for seasoning.

Spread the breadcrumb mixture to the salmon.

Bake the salmon for 15 to 20 minutes, or until it's cooked through.

Nutritional Facts about (per serving):

280 calories

125 milligrams of sodium

500 milligrams of potassium

23 g of protein

200 milligrams of phosphorus

22. *Chicken and Vegetable Stir-Fry*

Prep Time: 15 minutes

Cooking Time: 20 minutes

Servings: 4

Ingredients:

2 chicken breasts, sliced

2 tablespoons of gluten-free soy sauce

1 tablespoon of sesame oil

1 bell pepper, sliced

1 cup broccoli florets

1 carrot, sliced

1 onion, chopped

2 cloves garlic, minced

1 teaspoon of grated ginger

Directions:

Chicken should be marinated in soy sauce for ten minutes in a bowl.

In a wok or big skillet, heat up the sesame oil over medium-high heat.

Stir-fry the chicken until it's done and then set it aside.

Stir-fry the bell pepper, broccoli, carrot, onion, garlic, and ginger in the same wok until the veggies are crisp-tender.

Stir thoroughly to blend the chicken after returning it to the wok.

Nutritional Facts (per serving):

220 calories

300 mg of sodium

400 mg of potassium and 26 g of protein

220 milligrams of phosphorus

23. Grilled Vegetable Kabobs

Prep Time: 15 minutes (plus marinating time)

Cooking Time: 10 minutes

Servings: 4

Ingredients:

1 zucchini, cut into chunks

1 bell pepper, cut into chunks

1 red onion, cut into chunks

8 cherry tomatoes

1/4 cup olive oil

2 tablespoons of balsamic vinegar

1 tablespoon of chopped fresh basil

Salt and pepper to taste

Directions:

Mix the olive oil, balsamic vinegar, basil, salt, and pepper in a big sized bowl.

After adding the veggies to the marinade, give it at least half an hour to marinate.

Thread the vegetables on skewers.

For about ten minutes, grill over medium heat, rotating regularly.

Nutritional Facts (per serving):

150 calories

25 milligrams of sodium

350 mg of potassium and 2 g of protein

50 milligrams of phosphorus

24. Stuffed Acorn Squash

Prep Time: 15 minutes

Cooking Time: 45 minutes

Servings: 4

Ingredients:

2 acorn squashes, halved and seeded

1 cup quinoa, rinsed

2 cups vegetable broth

1/2 cup dried cranberries

1/2 cup chopped pecans

1/2 cup chopped parsley

1/4 cup olive oil

Salt and pepper to taste

Directions:

Turn the oven on to 375°F, or 190°C.

Squash halves should be placed cut-side up on a baking pan. Add a drizzle of olive oil and season with pepper and salt. Bake for twenty-five minutes.

Follow the directions on the package to boil the quinoa in vegetable stock in a saucepan.

Cooked quinoa should be combined with parsley, pecans, and cranberries.

After adding the quinoa mixture to the squash halves, bake for an additional 20 minutes.

Nutritional Facts (per serving):

330 calories

150 milligrams of sodium

500 milligrams of potassium

Six grams of protein

150 milligrams of phosphorus

25. *Creamy Mushroom Risotto*

Prep Time: 10 minutes

Cooking Time: 25 minutes

Servings: 4

Ingredients:

1 cup arborio rice

3 cups low-sodium chicken or vegetable broth

1 onion, chopped

2 cups sliced mushrooms

2 cloves garlic, minced

1/4 cup grated Parmesan cheese

2 tablespoons of olive oil

Salt and pepper to taste

Directions:

Heat up the olive oil in a big skillet over medium heat.

Add the garlic and onion, and cook until transparent.

Cook the mushrooms until they become tender.

Add arborio rice and let it cook for a minute.

One cup of broth at a time, gradually add it, stirring continuously until the liquid is absorbed before adding more.

Add the Parmesan cheese after the rice is soft and creamy. Add pepper and salt for seasoning.

Nutritional Facts (per serving):

300 calories

150 milligrams of sodium

250 milligrams of potassium

8 g of protein

180 milligrams of phosphorus

26. *Cauliflower Fried Rice*

Prep Time: 15 minutes

Cooking Time: 10 minutes

Servings: 4

Ingredients:

1 head cauliflower, grated

2 eggs, beaten

1 cup mixed vegetables (peas, carrots, corn)

2 tbsp gluten-free soy sauce

1 onion, chopped

1 clove garlic, minced

2 tablespoons of sesame oil

Directions:

heat the Sesame oil over medium heat in a big skillet.

Add the garlic and onion and sauté until tender.

For three minutes, add the mixed vegetables and simmer.

Add the soy sauce and grated cauliflower and stir.

Cook, stirring often, for 5 minutes.

After pushing the cauliflower mixture to one side of the skillet, cover the other side with the beaten eggs.

Add scrambled eggs to the cauliflower mixture.

Nutritional Facts (per serving):

180 calories

350 mg of sodium

450 milligrams of potassium

8 g of protein

120 milligrams of phosphorus

27. Beef and Broccoli

Prep Time: 15 minutes (plus marinating time)

Cooking Time: 10 minutes

Servings: 4

Ingredients:

1 lb beef sirloin, thinly sliced

1/4 cup gluten-free soy sauce

2 tablespoons of brown sugar

1 tablespoon of cornstarch

1 tablespoon of ginger, grated

2 cloves garlic, minced

2 cups broccoli florets

2 tablespoons of sesame oil

Directions:

Mix the soy sauce, brown sugar, cornstarch, ginger, and garlic in a bowl.

Give the steak a good marinating for at least half an hour.

In a big skillet, warm up the sesame oil over medium-high heat.

When the broccoli is crisp-tender, add it and remove it from the skillet.

Cook the beef in the skillet until it turns brown.

Put the broccoli back in the skillet and toss it with the beef.

Warm up thoroughly.

Nutritional Facts (per serving):

250 calories

500 milligrams of sodium

400 milligrams of potassium

25 g of protein

200 milligrams of phosphorus

28. Spinach and Feta Stuffed Chicken

Prep Time: 20 minutes

Cooking Time: 30 minutes

Servings: 4

Ingredients:

4 boneless, skinless chicken breasts

2 cups fresh spinach leaves

1/2 cup feta cheese, crumbled

1/4 cup sun-dried tomatoes, chopped

2 tablespoons of olive oil

Salt and pepper to taste

Directions:

Set the oven to 375°F, or 190°C.

On each of the chicken breasts, cut a pocket.

Place sun-dried tomatoes, feta, and spinach inside each.

Add the pepper and salt for seasoning.

Heat the olive oil in a pan over medium heat.

Sear chicken till browned on both sides.

Place the chicken in the oven and bake it for 20 minutes, or until it is thoroughly done.

Nutritional Facts (per serving):

290 calories

320 mg of sodium

300 milligrams of potassium

28 g of protein

220 milligrams of phosphorus

29. *Baked Lemon Herb Chicken*

Prep Time: 15 minutes

Cooking Time: 30 minutes

Servings: 4

Ingredients:

4 boneless chicken breasts

2 lemons, juiced and zested

3 cloves garlic, minced

2 tablespoons of olive oil

1 teaspoon dried thyme

1 teaspoon dried rosemary

Salt and pepper to taste

Directions:

Set the oven to 375°F, or 190°C.

Combine the lemon zest and juice, garlic, olive oil, rosemary, thyme, and salt & pepper in a bowl.

Transfer the chicken to a baking dish and cover with the mixture.

Bake the chicken for about 30 minutes, or until it is cooked through.

Nutritional Facts:

220 calories

70 mg of sodium

340 mg of potassium and 25 g of protein

200 milligrams of phosphorus

30. Grilled Salmon with Asparagus

Prep Time: 10 minutes

Cooking Time: 20 minutes

Servings: 4

Ingredients:

4 salmon fillets

1 bunch asparagus, trimmed

2 tbsp olive oil

1 lemon, sliced

Salt and pepper to taste

Directions:

Grill at a medium-high temperature.

Add salt and pepper to the fish and asparagus after brushing them with olive oil.

Grill asparagus and salmon for ten minutes on each side.

Serve with slices of lemon.

Facts about Nutrition:

300 calories

60 milligrams of sodium

500 milligrams of potassium

23 g of protein

250 milligrams of phosphorus

31. *Baked Apple Chips*

Prep Time: 10 minutes

Cooking Time: 2 hours

Servings: 4

Ingredients:

2 large apples, thinly sliced

1 teaspoon cinnamon

Directions:

Set the oven to a temperature of 200°F, or 95°C.

Place apple slices in an arrangement on a baking sheet and dust with cinnamon.

Bake until dried out, turning halfway through the two hours.

Nutritional Facts:

50 calories

Sodium: n/a

Potassium: one hundred milligrams

0.5 g of protein

10 milligrams of phosphorus

32. Carrot and Cucumber Sticks with Hummus

Prep Time: 10 minutes
Cooking Time: 0 minutes
Servings: 4

Ingredients:

2 big carrots, peeled and cut into sticks

1 cucumber, cut into sticks

1 cup hummus

Directions:

Serve the carrot and cucumber sticks alongside a hummus side for dunks.

Facts about Nutrition:

130 calories

200 milligrams of sodium

250 mg of potassium and 6 g of protein

120 milligrams of phosphorus

33. *Avocado and Gluten-Free Rice Cakes*

Prep Time: 5 minutes

Cooking Period: 0 Minutes

Servings: 2

Ingredients:

Two gluten-free rice cakes

One ripe avocado

Salt and pepper to taste

Lemon juice (optional)

Directions:

Spread the avocado mash over the rice cakes.

Add some salt and pepper for seasoning.

Add a squeeze of lemon juice

Nutritional Facts:

140 calories

30 milligrams of sodium

450 milligrams of potassium

2 g of protein

50 milligrams of phosphorus

34. Greek Yogurt with Berries and Honey

Prep Time: 5 minutes

Cooking Time: 0 minutes

Servings: 2

Ingredients:

1 cup plain Greek yogurt

1/2 cup mixed berries (strawberries, blueberries, raspberries)

1 tablespoon of honey

Directions:

Add berries to the top of Greek yogurt.

Pour some honey over it.

Nutritional Facts:

120 calories

45 milligrams of sodium

Protein: 10 g

Potassium: 200 mg

150 milligrams of phosphorus

35. *Cottage Cheese with Pineapple*

Prep Time: 5 minutes

Cooking Time: 0 minutes

Servings: 2

Ingredients:

1 cup low-fat cottage cheese

1/2 cup chopped pineapple

Directions:

Combine diced pineapple with cottage cheese.

Nutritional Facts:

110 calories

350 mg of sodium

180 mg potassium and 14 g protein

120 milligrams of phosphorus

36. Almond Butter on Gluten-Free Toast

Prep Time: 5 minutes

Cooking Time: 2 minutes

Servings: 2

Ingredients:

Two pieces of gluten-free bread

Two tablespoons of almond butter

Directions:

Bake the gluten-free bread.

Toast with almond butter spread on it.

Nutritional Facts:

210 calories

180 milligrams of sodium

150 mg of potassium and 5 g of protein

120 milligrams of phosphorus

37. Chia Seed Pudding:

Prep Time: 10 minutes (plus chilling)

Cooking Period: 0 minutes

Servings: 2

Ingredient:

One-fourth cup of chia seeds

One cup of almond milk

One tablespoon of maple syrup

Half a teaspoon vanilla extract

Use fresh fruit as a garnish (optional).

Directions:

In a dish, stir together chia seeds, almond milk, maple syrup, and vanilla extract.

Place in the refrigerator for four hours or overnight.

Garnish with fresh fruit and serve chilled.

Nutritional Facts:

150 calories

30 milligrams of sodium

Protein: 4 g; Potassium: 100 mg

200 milligrams of phosphorus

38. Roasted Chickpeas

Prep Time: 5 minutes

Cooking Time: 30 minutes

Servings: 4

Ingredients:

1 can (15 oz) chickpeas, drained and rinsed

1 tablespoon of olive oil

1/2 teaspoon salt

1/4 teaspoon black pepper

1/2 teaspoon paprika (optional)

Directions:

Set the oven to a temperature of 400°F, or 200°C.

Using a paper towel to pat dry the chickpeas, remove any loose skins.

Add paprika, salt, pepper, and olive oil to the chickpeas and toss.

Place onto a baking sheet and bake until crispy, stirring every 30 minutes.

Nutritional Information:

120 calories

300 mg of sodium

Protein: 5 g; Potassium: 200 mg

100 milligrams of phosphorus

39. *Veggie Sticks with Gluten-Free Ranch Dip*

Prep Time: 10 minutes

Cooking Time: 0 minutes

Servings: 4

Ingredients:

1/2 cup plain Greek yogurt

1 tablespoons of ranch seasoning mix (gluten-free)

Assorted veggies (carrots, celery, bell peppers), cut into sticks.

Directions

Mix the ranch seasoning with Greek yogurt.

Serve with a selection of dipping veggie sticks.

Nutritional Information:

35 calories

150 milligrams of sodium

180 mg potassium and 3 g protein

60 milligrams of phosphorus

40. Banana and Peanut Butter Roll-Ups

Prep Time: 5 minutes

Cooking Time: 0 minutes

Servings: 2

Ingredients:

2 medium bananas

2 tbsp peanut butter (gluten-free)

2 gluten-free tortillas

Directions:

Evenly distribute peanut butter over the tortillas.

Each tortilla should have a banana on it. Roll it up tightly.

Cut into pieces that are bite-sized.

Nutritional information:

210 calories

200 milligrams of sodium

400 mg of potassium and 5 proteins

41. *Flourless Chocolate Cake*

Prep Time: 15 minutes

Cooking Time: 25 minutes

Servings: 8

Ingredients:

4 ounces fine-quality bittersweet chocolate

1/2 cup unsalted butter

3/4 cup sugar

3 large eggs

1/2 cup unsweetened cocoa powder

Directions:

Set the oven to 375°F, or 190°C. An 8-inch circular cake pan should be greased.

In a double boiler, melt butter and chocolate together. Blend until silky.

Take off the heat, then thoroughly mix in the sugar. Whisk once more after adding the eggs.

Over the chocolate, sift the cocoa powder and stir until barely incorporated.

After adding the batter to the pan, bake it for about 25 minutes.

Nutritional Facts (Per serving):

280 calories

60 milligrams of sodium

150 milligrams of potassium

4 g of protein

100 milligrams of phosphorus

42. Almond and Coconut Macaroons

Prep Time: 15 minutes

Cooking Time: 15 minutes

Servings: 12

Ingredients:

1 3/4 cups shredded unsweetened coconut

3 large egg whites

1/2 cup sugar

1/2 cup almond flour

1 teaspoon vanilla extract

Directions:

Set the oven to 325°F, or 165°C.

Use parchment paper to line a baking sheet.

Beat the egg whites with the sugar. Add vanilla, coconut, and almond flour and stir.

Spoon batter onto the baking sheet in tablespoon amounts.

Bake for about 15 minutes, or until golden. Allow to cool.

Nutritional Facts (per Serving):

120 calories

35 milligrams of sodium

80 mg of potassium and 2 g of protein

40 milligrams of phosphorus

43. Gluten-Free Lemon Bars

Prep Time: 20 minutes

Cooking Time: 45 minutes

Servings: 9

Ingredients:

For the crust:

1 cup gluten-free flour blend

1/2 cup unsalted butter, melted

1/4 cup powdered sugar

For the filling:

2 large eggs

1 cup granulated sugar

2 tablespoons of gluten-free flour blend

1/4 cup lemon juice

Directions:

Set Your oven temperature to 175°C/350°F.

For the crust, combine flour, butter, and powdered sugar.

Press into a 9.5-inch square pan with it.

For 20 minutes, bake the crust.

Mix the ingredients for the filling and pour it over the baked crust.

Add another 25 minutes of baking. Once cooled, sprinkle with powdered sugar.

Nutritional Facts (per serving):

280 calories

70 mg of sodium

30 milligrams of potassium

3 g of protein

40 milligrams of phosphorus

44. *Baked Pears with Honey and Cinnamon*

Prep Time: 10 minutes

Cooking Time: 30 minutes

Servings: 4

Ingredients:

2 large ripe pears, halved and cored

2 tablespoons of honey

1/2 teaspoon of ground cinnamon

Directions:

Set your oven temperature to 175°C/350°F.

Halve the pears and place them cut-side up on a baking pan.

Sprinkle with cinnamon and drizzle with honey.

Bake for about 30 minutes, or until pears are soft.

Nutritional Facts (per half pear):

110 calories

Sodium: n/a

Potassium: one hundred milligrams

0.5 g of protein

10 milligrams of phosphorus

45. Gluten-Free Rice Pudding

Prep Time: 5 minutes

Cooking Time: 45 minutes

Servings: 6

Ingredients:

1/2 cup uncooked white rice

4 cups milk (or dairy-free alternative)

1/3 cup sugar

1/4 teaspoon of salt

1 teaspoon of vanilla extract

Directions:

In a saucepan, combine rice, milk, sugar, and salt; bring to a boil.

For about 45 minutes, or until the rice is cooked, reduce heat and simmer, stirring frequently.

Take off the heat and mix in the vanilla. Serve hot or cold.

Nutritional Facts (per serving):

190 calories

125 milligrams of sodium

150 mg of potassium and 5 g of protein

100 milligrams of phosphorus

46. No-Bake Peanut Butter Oat Bars

Prep Time: 15 minutes

Cooking Time: 0 minutes (chill time: 1 hour)

Servings: 10

Ingredients:

1 cup peanut butter (gluten-free)

1/2 cup honey

2 cups gluten-free rolled oats

Directions:

In a skillet over low heat, melt the peanut butter and honey together.

Add oats and stir until evenly coated.

Fill an 8 × 8-inch baking pan with mixture and press it in.

After an hour of refrigeration, cut into bars.

Nutritional Facts (per bar):

230 calories

100 milligrams of sodium

150 milligrams of potassium

Six grams of protein

120 milligrams of phosphorus

47. *Avocado Chocolate Mousse*

Prep Time: 10 minutes
Cooking Time: 0 minutes
Servings: 4

Ingredients:

2 ripe avocados, peeled and pitted

1/4 cup cocoa powder

1/4 cup honey or maple syrup

1/2 teaspoon of vanilla extract

Pinch of salt

Directions:

Add all ingredients into a food processor and blend. Process till it becomes smooth.

Let it cool for a minimum of half an hour before serving.

Nutritional Facts (per serving):

200 calories

20 milligrams of sodium

400 milligrams of potassium

3 g of protein

60 milligrams of phosphorus

48. Gluten-Free Apple Crisp

Prep Time: 15 minutes

Cooking Time: 45 minutes

Servings: 6

Ingredients:

4 medium apples, peeled and sliced

1/2 cup almond flour

1/2 cup gluten-free oats

1/3 cup brown sugar

1/4 cup butter, melted

1 tsp cinnamon

1/4 teaspoon nutmeg

Directions:

Set your oven temperature to 175°C/350°F.

Apple slices should be put in a baking dish.

Combine almond flour, oats, butter, brown sugar, cinnamon, and nutmeg in a bowl.

Over the apples, scatter the mixture.

Bake for 45 minutes, or until the apples are soft and the top is golden brown.

Facts about nutrition (per serving):

220 calories

55 milligrams of sodium

150 mg of potassium and 3 g of protein

60 milligrams of phosphorus

49. Chocolate-Dipped Strawberries

Prep Time: 15 minutes

Cooking Time: 0 minutes (chill time: 30 minutes)

Servings: 4

Ingredients:

12 large strawberries

4 oz gluten-free dark chocolate

1 tsp coconut oil

Directions:

In a double boiler or microwave, melt the dark chocolate and coconut oil together.

Place each strawberry on a dish lined with parchment after dipping it into the chocolate.

Chill for around half an hour or until the chocolate solidifies.

Nutritional Facts (for three strawberries per serving):

150 calories

20 milligrams of sodium

200 milligrams of potassium

2 g of protein

70 milligrams of phosphorus

50. Gluten-Free Blueberry Muffins

Prep Time: 10 minutes

Cooking Time: 25 minutes

Servings: 12 muffins

Ingredients:

2 cups gluten-free flour blend

1/2 cup sugar

1 tablespoon baking powder

1/2 teaspoon salt

1 cup almond milk

1/3 cup vegetable oil

1 egg

1 teaspoon vanilla extract

1 cup fresh blueberries

Directions:

Turn the oven on to 375°F, or 190°C. Use paper liners to line a muffin tray.

Mix the flour, sugar, baking powder, and salt in a bowl.

Mix the almond milk, oil, egg, and vanilla in a separate bowl.

Stir together the dry and wet ingredients; stir in the blueberries.

When a toothpick inserted into a muffin cup comes out clean, bake for 25 minutes.

Nutritional Facts (per muffin):

180 calories

150 milligrams of sodium

50 mg of potassium and 2 g of protein

90 milligrams of phosphorus

FREE: BONUS

7 day Meal Plan

Day 1

Breakfast: Greek Yogurt with Berries and Honey

Lunch: Quinoa & Vegetable Stuffed Peppers

Dinner: Baked Lemon Herb Chicken with Steamed Vegetables

Snack: Carrot and Cucumber Sticks with Hummus

Dessert: Flourless Chocolate Cake (small portion)

Day 2

Breakfast: Gluten-Free Blueberry Muffins

Lunch: Lentil Soup with Spinach

Dinner: Grilled Salmon with Asparagus

Snack: Baked Apple Chips

Dessert: Baked Pears with Honey and Cinnamon

Day 3

Breakfast: Scrambled Eggs with Gluten-Free Toast
Lunch: Vegetable Stir-Fry with Tofu
Dinner: Quinoa Stuffed Acorn Squash
Snack: Almond Butter on Gluten-Free Toast
Dessert: Chocolate-Dipped Strawberries

Day 4

Breakfast: Omelet with Spinach and Mushrooms
Lunch: Zucchini Noodles with Tomato Sauce
Dinner: Gluten-Free Lemon Bars
Snack: Gluten-Free Rice Cakes with Avocado
Dessert: Avocado Chocolate Mousse

Day 5

Breakfast: Smoothie with Banana, Almond Milk, and Gluten-Free Oats

Lunch: Grilled Chicken Salad with Olive Oil and Lemon Dressing

Dinner: Baked Cod with Lemon and Dill, with Roasted Sweet Potatoes

Snack: No-Bake Peanut Butter Oat Bars

Dessert: Almond and Coconut Macaroons

Day 6

Breakfast: Fruit Salad with a Dollop of Greek Yogurt

Lunch: Roasted Vegetable Quinoa Salad

Dinner: Chia Seed Pudding with Fresh Fruit

Snack: Roasted Chickpeas

Dessert: Gluten-Free Apple Crisp

Day 7

Breakfast: Gluten-Free Pancakes with Maple Syrup

Lunch: Tomato and Basil Soup

Dinner: Baked Cod with Lemon and Dill, served with a side of roasted sweet potatoes

Snack: Cottage Cheese with Pineapple

Dessert: Gluten-Free Rice Pudding

CONCLUSION

As we come to the end of this Gluten-free cookbook for seniors, let use this opportunity to congratulate for taking steps to improve your health and well-being using nutrition.

Care has been taken to make relevant dietary information available to help you make informed decisions regarding your recipes preparations and meal plan.

Use this guide. Implement the recipes and watch your health blossom for good

Congratulations

Made in United States
Troutdale, OR
03/07/2024

18277411R00046